National Cancer Institute

Understanding Prostate Changes

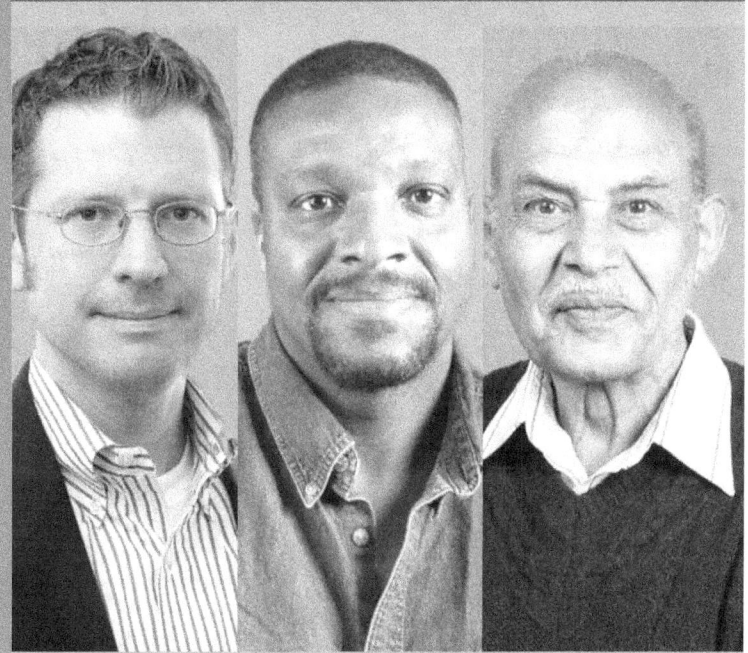

A Health Guide for Men

U.S. DEPARTMENT OF HEALTH AND HUMAN SERVICES

National Institutes of Health

Table of Contents

Introduction to the Prostate

You may be reading this booklet because you are having prostate problems. The booklet can help answer your questions about prostate changes, such as:

- What are common prostate changes?

- How are these changes treated?

- What do I need to know about testing for prostate changes, including cancer?

This booklet can give you basic information about common prostate changes. If you are making decisions about **prostate cancer** treatment, there are other resources available. See the "For More Information" section on page 29.

Important words are in **bold**, and their meanings are listed in the "Words to Know" section on page 31.

What is the prostate?

The **prostate** is a small gland in men. It is part of the male **reproductive system**.

The prostate is about the size and shape of a walnut. It sits low in the **pelvis**, below the **bladder** and just in front of the **rectum**. The prostate helps make **semen**, the milky fluid that carries **sperm** from the **testicles** through the **penis** when a man **ejaculates**.

The prostate surrounds part of the **urethra**, a tube that carries **urine** out of the bladder and through the penis.

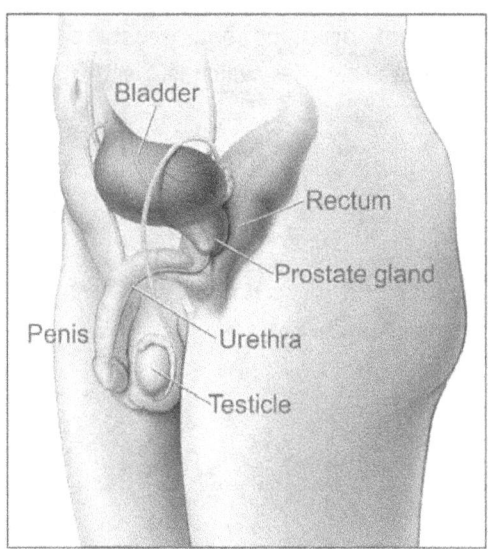

How does the prostate change as you get older?

Because the prostate gland tends to grow larger with age, it may squeeze the urethra and cause problems in passing urine. Sometimes men in their 30s and 40s may begin to have these urinary **symptoms** and need medical attention. For others, symptoms aren't noticed until much later in life. An **infection** or a **tumor** can also make the prostate larger. Be sure to tell your doctor if you have any of the **urinary** symptoms listed below.

Tell your doctor if you have these urinary symptoms:

- Are passing urine more during the day

- Have an urgent need to pass urine

- Have less urine flow

- Feel burning when you pass urine

- Need to get up many times during the night to pass urine

What prostate changes should you be aware of?

Growing older raises your risk of prostate problems. The three most common prostate problems are:

- Inflammation (**prostatitis**)
- Enlarged prostate (**BPH**, or **benign prostatic hyperplasia**)
- Prostate cancer

One change does not lead to another. For example, having prostatitis or an enlarged prostate does not increase your risk of prostate cancer. It is also possible for you to have more than one condition at the same time.

Most prostate changes are <u>not</u> cancer.

Prostate Changes That Are Not Cancer

What is prostatitis and how is it treated?

Prostatitis is an **inflammation** of the prostate gland that may result from a bacterial infection. It affects at least half of all men at some time during their lives. Having this condition does not increase your risk of any other prostate disease.

Prostatitis Symptoms

- Trouble passing urine

- A burning or stinging feeling or pain when passing urine

- Strong, frequent urge to pass urine, even when there is only a small amount of urine

- Chills and high fever

- Low back pain or body aches

- Pain low in the belly, in the **groin**, or behind the **scrotum**

- **Rectal** pressure or pain

- Urethral **discharge** with bowel movements

- **Genital** and rectal throbbing

- Sexual problems and loss of sex drive

- Painful **ejaculation** (sexual climax)

Several tests, such as DRE and a urine test, can be done to see if you have prostatitis. Correct diagnosis of your exact type of prostatitis is key to getting the best treatment. Even if you have no symptoms you should follow your doctor's advice to complete treatment.

There are four types of prostatitis:

▧ Acute bacterial prostatitis

This type is caused by a **bacterial** infection and comes on suddenly (**acute**). Symptoms include severe chills and fever. There is often blood in the urine. Your PSA level (see "**PSA test**" on page 24) may be higher than normal. You must go to the doctor's office or emergency room for treatment. It's the least common of the four types, yet it's the easiest to diagnose and treat.

Treatment: Most cases can be cured with a high dose of **antibiotics**, taken for 7 to 14 days, and then lower doses for several weeks. You may also need drugs to help with pain or discomfort. If your PSA level was high, it will likely return to normal once the infection is cleared up.

▧ Chronic bacterial prostatitis

Also caused by bacteria, this type of prostatitis doesn't come on suddenly, but it can be bothersome. The only symptom you may have is bladder infections that keep coming back. The cause may be a defect in the prostate that lets bacteria collect in the **urinary tract**.

Treatment: Antibiotic treatment over a longer period of time is best for this type. Treatment lasts from 4 to 12 weeks. This type of treatment clears up about 60 percent of cases. Long-term, low-dose antibiotics may help relieve symptoms in cases that won't clear up.

■ Chronic prostatitis/chronic pelvic pain syndrome

This disorder is the most common but least understood type of prostatitis. Found in men of any age from late teens to the elderly, its symptoms can come and go without warning. There can be pain or discomfort in the groin or bladder area. Infection-fighting cells are often present, even though no bacteria can be found.

Treatment: There are several different treatments for this problem, based on your symptoms. These include anti-inflammatory medications and other pain control treatments, such as warm baths. Other medicines, such as **alpha-blockers**, may also be given. Alpha-blockers relax muscle **tissue** in the prostate to make passing urine easier. Some men are treated with antibiotics in case the symptoms are caused by an undetected infection.

■ Asymptomatic inflammatory prostatitis

You don't have symptoms with this condition. It is often found when you are undergoing tests for other conditions, such as to determine the cause of infertility or to look for prostate cancer. If you have this form of prostatitis, your PSA test (see "PSA test" on page 24) may show a higher number than normal.

Treatment: Men with this condition are usually not treated, but a repeat PSA test will usually be done if the PSA number is high.

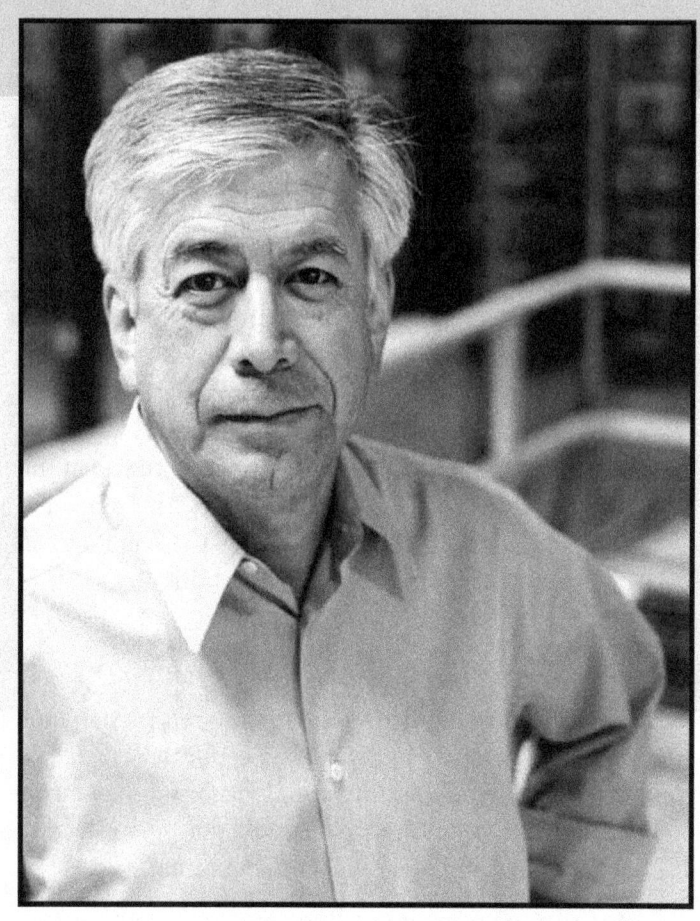

"Changes happen so slowly that you don't even realize they're happening."

What is enlarged prostate or BPH?

BPH stands for benign prostatic hyperplasia.

Benign means "not cancer," and **hyperplasia** means abnormal cell growth. The result is that the prostate becomes enlarged. BPH is not linked to cancer and does not increase your risk of getting prostate cancer—yet the symptoms for BPH and prostate cancer can be similar.

BPH Symptoms

BPH symptoms usually start after the age of 50. They can include:

- Trouble starting a urine stream or making more than a dribble
- Passing urine often, especially at night
- Feeling that the bladder has not fully emptied
- A strong or sudden urge to pass urine
- Weak or slow urine stream
- Stopping and starting again several times while passing urine
- Pushing or straining to begin passing urine

At its worst, BPH can lead to:

- A weak bladder
- Backflow of urine, causing bladder or **kidney** infections
- Complete block in the flow of urine
- Kidney failure

BPH affects most men as they get older. It can lead to urinary problems like those with prostatitis. BPH rarely causes symptoms before age 40, but more than half of men in their 60s and most men in their 70s and 80s will have signs of BPH.

The prostate gland is about the size of a walnut when a man is in his 20s. By the time he is 40, it may have grown slightly larger, to the size of an apricot. By age 60, it may be the size of a lemon.

The enlarged prostate can press against the bladder and the urethra. This can slow down or block urine flow. Some men might find it hard to start a urine stream, even though they feel the need to go. Once the urine stream has started, it may be hard to stop. Other men may feel like they need to pass urine all the time, or they are awakened during sleep with the sudden need to pass urine.

Early BPH symptoms take many years to turn into bothersome problems. These early symptoms are a cue to see your doctor.

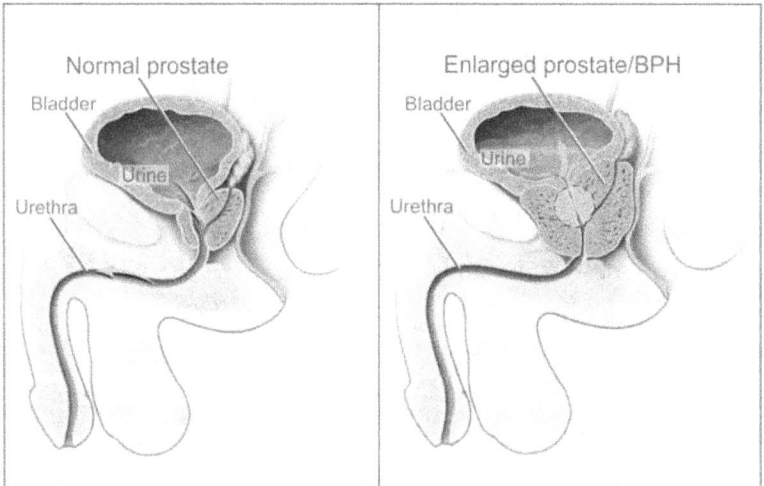

Urine flow in a normal (left) and enlarged (right) prostate. In diagram on the left, urine flows freely. On the right, urine flow is affected because the enlarged prostate is pressing on the bladder and urethra.

How is BPH treated?

Some men with BPH eventually find their symptoms to be bothersome enough to need treatment. BPH cannot be cured, but drugs or **surgery** can often relieve its symptoms.

There are three ways to manage BPH:

- **Watchful waiting** (regular follow-up with your doctor)

- Drug therapy

- Surgery

Talk with your doctor about the best choice for you. Your symptoms may change over time, so be sure to tell your doctor about any new changes.

Watchful waiting

Men with mild symptoms of BPH who do not find them bothersome often choose this approach.

Watchful waiting means getting annual check-ups. The check-ups can include DREs and other tests (see "Types of Tests" on page 23). Treatment is started only when the symptoms become too much of a problem.

If you choose watchful waiting, these simple steps may help lessen your symptoms:

- Limit drinking in the evening, especially drinks with **alcohol** or **caffeine**.

- Empty your bladder all the way when you pass urine.

- Use the restroom often. Don't wait for long periods without passing urine.

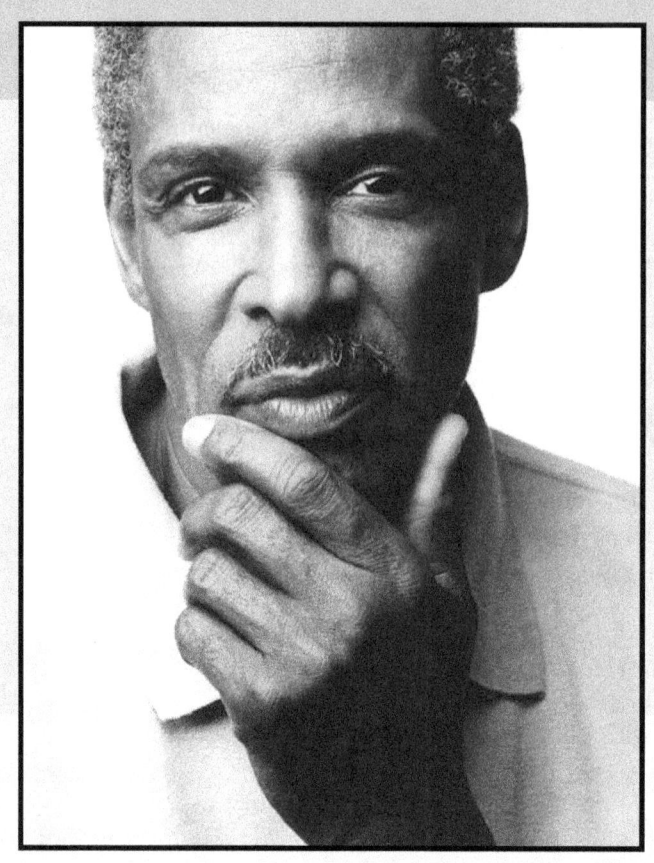

"My doctor and I decide visit by visit about how long I should stay on watchful waiting for my BPH."

Some medications can make BPH symptoms worse, so talk with your doctor or pharmacist about any medicines you are taking, such as:

- **Over-the-counter** cold and cough medicines (especially **antihistamines**)
- Tranquilizers
- **Antidepressants**
- **Blood pressure** medicine

Your doctor may be able to prescribe other medication that does not increase BPH symptoms.

Drug therapy

Many American men with mild to moderate BPH symptoms have chosen **prescription** drugs over surgery since the early 1990s. Two main types of drugs are used. One type relaxes muscles near the prostate, and the other type shrinks the prostate gland. Some evidence shows that taking both drugs together may work best to keep BPH symptoms from getting worse.

Alpha-blockers

These drugs (see the table on page 14) help relax muscles near the prostate to relieve pressure and let urine flow more freely, but they don't shrink the size of the prostate. For many men, these drugs can improve urine flow and reduce the symptoms of BPH within days. Possible **side effects** include dizziness, headache, and fatigue.

5-alpha reductase inhibitors

These drugs (see the table on page 14) help shrink the prostate. They relieve symptoms by blocking the activity of an **enzyme** known as 5-alpha reductase. This enzyme changes the male hormone **testosterone** into **dihydrotestosterone** (DHT), which stimulates prostate growth. When the action of 5-alpha reductase is blocked, DHT production is lowered and prostate growth slows.

This helps shrink the prostate, reduce blockage, and limit the need for surgery.

Taking these drugs can help increase urine flow and reduce your symptoms. You must continue to take these drugs to prevent symptoms from coming back.

5-alpha reductase inhibitors can cause the following side effects in a small percentage of men:

- Decreased interest in sex
- Trouble getting or keeping an **erection**
- Smaller amount of semen with ejaculation

It's important to note that taking these drugs may lower your PSA test number. There is also evidence that these drugs lower the risk of getting prostate cancer, but whether they can help lower the risk of dying from prostate cancer is still unclear.

BPH Medications			
Category	Activity	Generic Name	Brand Name
Alpha-blockers	Relax muscles near prostate	alfuzosin	Uroxatral
		doxazosin	Cardura
		silodosin	Rapaflo
		tamsulosin	Flomax
		terazosin	Hytrin
5-alpha reductase inhibitors	Slows prostate growth, shrinks prostate	finasteride	Proscar or Propecia
		dutasteride	Avodart

Surgery

The number of prostate surgeries has gone down over the years. But operations for BPH are still among the most common surgeries for American men. Surgery is used when symptoms are severe or drug therapy has not worked well.

Types of surgery for BPH include:

■ **TURP (transurethral resection of the prostate).** The most common surgery for BPH, TURP accounts for 90 percent of all BPH surgeries. The doctor passes an instrument through the urethra and trims away extra prostate tissue. A **spinal block (anesthesia)** is used to numb the area. Tissue is sent to the laboratory to check for prostate cancer.

TURP generally avoids the two main dangers linked to another type of surgery called open prostatectomy (complete removal of the prostate gland through a cut in the lower abdomen):

- **Incontinence** (not being able to hold in urine)
- **Impotence** (not being able to have an erection)

However, TURP can have serious side effects, such as bleeding. In addition, men may have to stay in the hospital and need a **catheter** for a few days after surgery.

■ **TUIP (transurethral incision of the prostate).** This surgery, which is similar to TURP, is used on slightly enlarged prostate glands. The surgeon places one or two small cuts in the prostate. This relieves pressure without trimming away tissue. It has a low risk of side effects. Like TURP, this treatment helps with urine flow by widening the urethra.

■ **TUNA (transurethral needle ablation).** Radio waves are used to burn away excess prostate tissue. TUNA helps with urine flow, relieves symptoms, and may have fewer side effects than TURP. Most men need a catheter to drain urine for a period of time after the procedure.

■ **TUMT (transurethral microwave thermotherapy).** Microwaves sent through a catheter are used to destroy excess prostate tissue. This can be an option for men who should not have major surgery because they have other medical problems.

■ **TUVP (transurethral electroevaporation of the prostate).** An electrical current is used to vaporize prostate tissue.

■ **Laser surgery.** The doctor passes a **laser** fiber through the urethra into the prostate, using a **cystoscope**, and then delivers several bursts of laser energy. The laser energy destroys prostate tissue and helps improve urine flow. Like TURP, laser surgery requires anesthesia. One advantage of laser surgery over TURP is that laser surgery causes little blood loss. The recovery period for laser surgery may be shorter too. However, laser surgery may not be effective on larger prostates.

■ **Open prostatectomy.** This may be the only option in rare cases, such as when the **obstruction** is severe, the prostate is very large, or other procedures can't be done. **General anesthesia** or a spinal block is used, and a catheter remains for 3 to 7 days after the surgery. This surgery carries the highest risk of **complications**. Tissue is sent to the laboratory to check for prostate cancer.

Be sure to discuss options with your doctor and ask about the potential short- and long-term benefits and risks with each procedure. For a list of questions to ask, see the "Checklist of Questions for Your Doctor" on page 28.

Prostate Cancer

Things to know

Prostate cancer means that cancer cells form in the tissues of the prostate. It is the most common cancer in American men after **skin cancer**.

Prostate cancer tends to grow slowly compared with most other cancers. Cell changes may begin 10, 20, or even 30 years before a tumor gets big enough to cause symptoms. Eventually, cancer cells may spread (**metastasize**) throughout the body. By the time symptoms appear, the cancer may already be advanced.

By age 50, very few men have symptoms of prostate cancer, yet some **precancerous** or cancer cells may be present. More than half of all American men have some cancer in their prostate glands by the age of 80. Most of these cancers never pose a problem. They may never cause symptoms or become a serious threat to health.

Most men with prostate cancer do not die from this disease.

- About 16 percent of American men are diagnosed with prostate cancer at some point in their lives.
- About 3 percent of American men will die of prostate cancer.

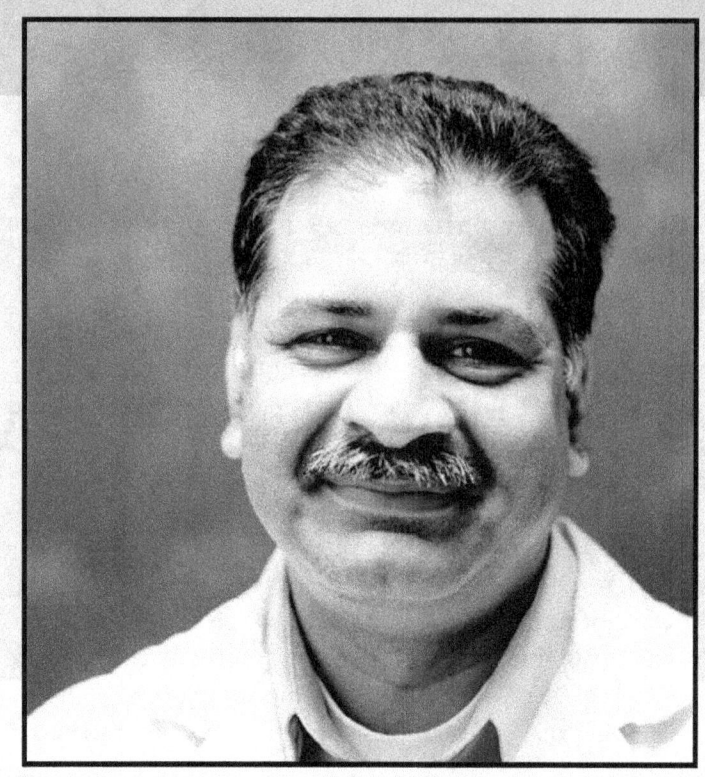

"When I first learned I might have a prostate problem, I was afraid it was cancer."

Symptoms

The symptoms of prostate cancer can be similar to the symptoms of BPH.

Prostate Cancer Symptoms

- Trouble passing urine
- Frequent urge to pass urine, especially at night
- Weak or interrupted urine stream
- Pain or burning when passing urine
- Blood in the urine or semen
- Painful ejaculation
- Nagging pain in the back, hips, or pelvis

Prostate cancer can spread to the **lymph nodes** of the pelvis. Or it may spread throughout the body. It tends to spread to the bones. So bone pain, especially in the back, can be a symptom of advanced prostate cancer.

Risk factors

Some **risk factors** have been linked to prostate cancer. A risk factor is something that can raise your chance of developing a disease. Having one or more risk factors doesn't mean that you will get prostate cancer. It just means that your risk of the disease is greater.

- Age. Men who are 50 or older have a higher risk of prostate cancer.

- Race. African-American men have the highest risk of prostate cancer—the disease tends to start at younger ages and grows faster than in men of other races. After African-American men, prostate cancer is most common among white men, followed by Hispanic and Native American men. Asian-American men have the lowest rates of prostate cancer.

■ **Family history.** Men whose fathers or brothers have had prostate cancer have a 2 to 3 times higher risk of prostate cancer than men who do not have a **family history** of the disease. A man who has 3 immediate family members with prostate cancer has about 10 times the risk of a man who does not have a family history of prostate cancer. The younger a man's relatives are when they have prostate cancer, the greater his risk for developing the disease. Prostate cancer risk also appears to be slightly higher for men from families with a history of **breast cancer**.

■ **Diet.** The risk of prostate cancer may be higher for men who eat high-fat diets.

Can prostate cancer be prevented?

Large research studies are looking at how prostate cancer can be prevented. Studies have shown that 5-alpha reductase inhibitors **finasteride** and **dutasteride** can lower the risk of developing prostate cancer, but whether they can decrease the risk of dying of prostate cancer is still unclear.

To find out more, see the "For More Information" section on page 29.

Prostate Cancer Screening

Screening means testing for cancer before you have any symptoms. A screening test may help find cancer at an early **stage**, when it is less likely to have spread and may be easier to treat. By the time symptoms appear, the cancer may have started to spread.

The most useful screening tests are those that have been proven to lower a person's risk of dying from cancer. Doctors do not yet know whether prostate cancer screening lowers the risk of dying from prostate cancer. Therefore, large research studies, with thousands of men, are now going on to study prostate cancer screening. The National Cancer Institute is studying the combination of PSA testing and DRE as a way to get more accurate results.

Although some people feel it is best to treat any cancer that is found, including cancers found through screening, prostate cancer treatment can cause serious and sometimes permanent side effects. Some doctors are concerned that many men whose cancer is detected by screening are being treated—and experiencing side effects—unnecessarily.

Talk with your doctor about your risk of prostate cancer and your need for screening tests.

Talking With Your Doctor

Different kinds of doctors and other health care professionals manage prostate health. They can help you find the best care, answer your questions, and address your concerns. These health care professionals include:

- Family doctors and internists

- Physician assistants (PAs) and nurse practitioners (NPs)

- **Urologists**, who are experts in diseases of the urinary tract system and the male reproductive system

- **Urologic oncologists**, who are experts in treating cancers of the urinary system and the male reproductive system

- **Radiation oncologists**, who use radiation therapy to treat cancer

- **Medical oncologists**, who treat cancer with medications such as hormone treatments and chemotherapy

- **Pathologists**, who identify diseases by studying cells and tissues under a microscope

View these professionals as your partners—expert advisors and helpers in your health care. Talking openly with your doctors can help you learn more about your prostate changes and the tests to expect.

It is a good idea to get a copy of your pathology report from your doctor and carry it with you as you talk with your health care providers.

Types of Tests

These types of tests are most often used to check the prostate:

Health history and current symptoms

This first step lets your doctor hear and understand the "story" of your prostate concerns. You'll be asked whether you have symptoms, how long you've had them, and how much they affect your lifestyle. Your **personal medical history** also includes any risk factors, pain, fever, or trouble passing urine. You may be asked to give a urine sample for testing.

Digital rectal exam (DRE)

DRE is a standard way to check the prostate. With a gloved and **lubricated** finger, your doctor feels the prostate from the rectum. The test lasts about 10-15 seconds.

This exam checks for:

- The size, firmness, and texture of the prostate
- Any hard areas, lumps, or growth spreading beyond the prostate
- Any pain caused by touching or pressing the prostate

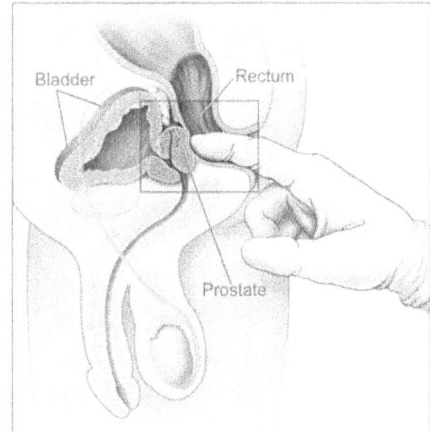

The DRE allows the doctor to feel only one side of the prostate. A PSA test is another way to help your doctor check the health of your prostate.

Prostate-specific antigen (PSA) test

The U.S. **Food and Drug Administration (FDA)** has approved the use of the PSA test along with a DRE to help detect prostate cancer in men age 50 and older.

PSA is a **protein** made by prostate cells. It is normally secreted into **ducts** in the prostate, where it helps make semen, but sometimes it leaks into the blood. When PSA is in the blood, it can be measured with a blood test called the PSA test.

In prostate cancer, more PSA gets into the blood than is normal. However, a high PSA blood level is not proof of cancer, and many other things can cause a **false-positive test result**. For example, blood PSA levels are often increased in men with prostatitis or BPH. Even things that disturb the prostate gland—such as riding a bicycle or motorcycle, or having a DRE, an **orgasm** within the past 24 hours, a prostate **biopsy**, or prostate surgery—may increase PSA levels.

Also, some prostate glands naturally produce more PSA than others. PSA levels go up with age. African-American men tend to have higher PSA levels in general than men of other races. And some drugs, such as finasteride and dutasteride, can cause a man's PSA level to go down.

PSA tests are often used to follow men after prostate cancer treatment to check for signs of cancer **recurrence**.

It is not yet known for certain whether PSA testing to screen for prostate cancer can reduce a man's risk of dying from the disease.

Researchers are working to learn more about:

- The PSA test's ability to help doctors tell the difference between prostate cancer and benign prostate problems
- The best thing to do if a man has a high PSA level

For now, men and their doctors use PSA readings over time as a guide to see if more follow-up is needed.

What do PSA results mean?

PSA levels are measured in terms of the amount of PSA per volume of fluid tested. Doctors often use a value of 4 **nanograms** (ng) or higher per milliliter of blood as a sign that further tests, such as a prostate biopsy, are needed.

Your doctor may monitor your PSA velocity, which means the rate of change in your PSA level over time. Rapid increases in PSA readings may suggest cancer. If you have a mildly elevated PSA level, you and your doctor may choose to do PSA tests on a scheduled basis and watch for any change in the PSA velocity.

Free PSA test

This test is used for men who have higher PSA levels. The standard PSA test measures total PSA, which includes both PSA that is attached, or bound, to other proteins and PSA that is free, or not bound. The free PSA test measures free PSA only. Free PSA is linked to benign prostate conditions, such as BPH, whereas bound PSA is linked to cancer. The percentage of free PSA can help tell what kind of prostate problem you have.

- If both total PSA and free PSA are higher than normal (high percentage of free PSA), this suggests BPH rather than cancer.

- If total PSA is high but free PSA is not (low percentage of free PSA), cancer is more likely. More testing, such as a biopsy, should be done.

You and your doctor should talk about your personal risk and free PSA results. Then you can decide together whether to have follow-up biopsies and, if so, how often.

Prostate biopsy

If your symptoms or test results suggest prostate cancer, your doctor will refer you to a specialist (a urologist) for a prostate biopsy. A biopsy is usually done in the doctor's office.

For a biopsy, small tissue samples are taken directly from the prostate. Your doctor will take samples from several areas of the prostate gland. This can help lower the chance of missing any areas of the gland that may have cancer cells. Like other cancers, prostate cancer can be diagnosed only by looking at tissue under a microscope.

Most men who have biopsies after prostate cancer screening exams do not have cancer.

If a biopsy is positive

A **positive test result** after a biopsy means prostate cancer is present. A pathologist will check your biopsy sample for cancer cells and will give it a **Gleason score**. The Gleason score ranges from 2 to 10 and describes how likely it is that a tumor will spread. The lower the number, the less **aggressive** the tumor is and the less likely it will spread.

"There is no magic PSA level below which a man can be assured of having no risk of prostate cancer or above which a biopsy should automatically be performed. A man's decision to have a prostate biopsy requires a thoughtful discussion with his physician, considering not only the PSA level, but also his other risk factors, his overall health status, and how he perceives the risks and benefits of early detection."

—Dr. Howard Parnes, Chief of the Prostate and Urologic Cancer Research Group, Division of Cancer Prevention, National Cancer Institute

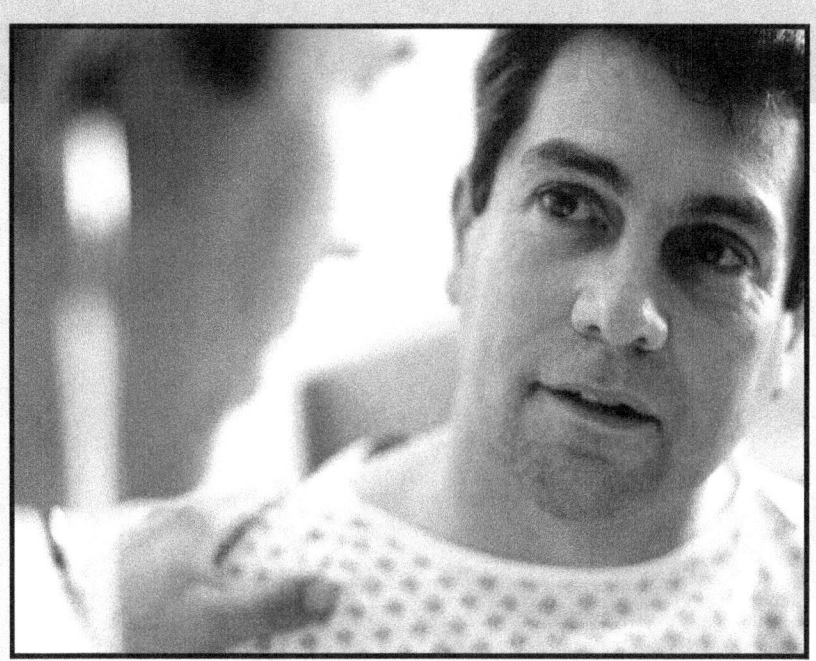

"While it's important to make your own decision about cancer screening, everybody should consider getting a second opinion before getting something like a biopsy."

Treatment options depend on the stage (or extent) of the cancer (stages range from 1 to 4), Gleason score, PSA level, and your age and general health. This information will be available from your doctor and is listed on your pathology report.

Reaching a decision about treatment of your prostate cancer is a complex process. Many men find it helpful to talk with their doctors, family, friends, and other men who have faced similar decisions.

Checklist of questions to ask your doctor

- ☐ What type of prostate problem do I have?

- ☐ Is more testing needed and what will it tell me?

- ☐ If I decide on watchful waiting, what changes in my symptoms should I look for and how often should I be tested?

- ☐ What type of treatment do you recommend for my prostate problem?

- ☐ For men like me, has this treatment worked?

- ☐ How soon would I need to start treatment and how long would it last?

- ☐ Do I need medicine and how long would I need to take it before seeing improvement in my symptoms?

- ☐ What are the side effects of the medicine?

- ☐ Are there other medicines that could interfere with this medication?

- ☐ If I need surgery, what are the benefits and risks?

- ☐ Would I have any side effects from surgery that could affect my quality of life?

- ☐ Are these side effects temporary or permanent?

- ☐ How long is recovery time after surgery?

- ☐ Will I be able to fully return to normal?

- ☐ How will this affect my sex life?

- ☐ How often should I visit the doctor to monitor my condition?

For More Information

National Cancer Institute

National Cancer Institute Services

NCI has comprehensive research-based information on cancer prevention, screening, diagnosis, treatment, genetics, and supportive care. We also have a clinical trials database and can offer tailored searches.

Web site ....www.cancer.gov and www.cancer.gov/espanol

Online Chat ....www.cancer.gov/livehelp

E-mail ....cancergovstaff@mail.nih.gov

Phone 1-800-4-CANCER (1-800-422-6237)

Publications ....www.cancer.gov/publications
or call 1-800-4-CANCER

Free resources to ask for include:

- *NCI Fact Sheet: Prostate-Specific Antigen (PSA) Test*
- *What You Need To Know About Prostate Cancer*
- *Treatment Choices for Men With Early-Stage Prostate Cancer*

We invite you to call or go online to talk with our trained information specialists, who speak English or Spanish, to:

- Get answers to any cancer-related questions you may have
- Get free NCI publications
- Learn more about specific resources and organizations in your area
- Find information on the NCI Web site, www.cancer.gov

Other Federal Resources

Centers for Disease Control and Prevention (CDC)

Phone 1-800-CDC-INFO (800-232-4636)

TTY 1-888-232-6348

E-mail ....cdcinfo@cdc.gov

Web site...............www.cdc.gov/cancer/prostate

Free booklets that are available include:

- *Prostate Cancer Screening: A Decision Guide*
- *Prostate Cancer Screening: A Decision Guide for African Americans*
- *La Detección del Cáncer de Próstata: Una Guía para Hispanos en los Estados Unidos*

Medicare

For information about Medicare benefits, contact:

Phone 1-800-MEDICARE (1-800-633-4227)

TTY 1-877-486-2048

Web site...............www.cms.hhs.gov

The National Institute of Diabetes and Digestive and Kidney Diseases (NIDDK)

NIDDK conducts and supports basic and clinical research on many of the most serious diseases affecting public health.

National Kidney and Urologic Diseases Information Clearinghouse is a service of NIDDK. They have free booklets on prostate problems, conditions, and research.

Phone 1-800-891-5390

Web site...............www.niddk.nih.gov

Words to Know

5-alpha reductase inhibitor: A drug that shrinks the prostate gland, used to treat BPH.

acute: Symptoms or signs that begin and get worse quickly. The opposite of acute is chronic.

aggressive: A quickly growing cancer.

alcohol: A chemical substance found in beer, wine, and liquor. Alcohol is also found in some medicines, mouthwashes, essential oils (scented liquid taken from plants), and household products.

alpha-blockers: Drugs that relax muscles in the prostate. Alpha-blockers are used to treat BPH.

anesthesia: A loss of feeling or awareness caused by drugs or other substances. Anesthesia keeps patients from feeling pain during surgery or other procedures. Local anesthesia is a loss of feeling in one small area of the body. Regional anesthesia is a loss of feeling in a part of the body, such as an arm or leg. General anesthesia is a loss of feeling and a complete loss of awareness that feels like a very deep sleep.

antibiotic: A drug used to treat infections caused by bacteria and other microorganisms.

antidepressants: Drugs used to treat depression.

antihistamine: A type of drug that blocks the action of histamines, which can cause fever, itching, sneezing, a runny nose, and watery eyes. Antihistamines are used to prevent fevers in patients receiving blood transfusions and to treat allergies, coughs, and colds.

asymptomatic: Having no signs or symptoms of disease.

bacteria: A large group of single-cell microorganisms. Some cause infections and disease in animals and humans. The singular of bacteria is bacterium.

benign: Not cancerous. Benign tumors do not spread to tissues around them or to other parts of the body.

biopsy: The removal of cells or tissues from the body for examination under a microscope. When doctors remove only a sample of tissue, it is called an incisional biopsy or core biopsy. When a whole tumor or lesion is removed, it is called an excisional biopsy. When doctors use a needle to remove a sample of tissue or fluid, it is called a needle biopsy or fine-needle biopsy.

bladder: The organ that stores urine.

blood pressure: The force of circulating blood on the walls of the arteries. Blood pressure is taken using two measurements: systolic (measured when the heart beats, when blood pressure is at its highest) and diastolic (measured between heart beats, when blood pressure is at its lowest). Blood pressure is written with the systolic blood pressure first, followed by the diastolic blood pressure (for example 120/80).

BPH (benign prostatic hyperplasia): A benign (not cancer) condition in which an overgrowth of prostate tissue pushes against the urethra and the bladder, blocking the flow of urine. Also called benign prostatic hypertrophy.

breast cancer: Cancer that forms in tissues of the breast, usually the ducts (tubes that carry milk to the nipple) and lobules (glands that make milk). It occurs in both men and women, although male breast cancer is rare.

caffeine: A substance found in the leaves and beans of the coffee tree, in tea, yerba mate, guarana berries, and in small amounts in cocoa. It can also be made in the laboratory, and is added to some soft drinks, foods, and medicines. Caffeine increases brain activity, alertness, attention, and energy. It may also increase blood pressure, heart rate, breathing rate, and the loss of water from the body in urine.

catheter: A flexible tube used to deliver fluids into or withdraw fluids from the body.

chronic: A disease or condition that stays bad or gets worse over a long period of time.

complication: In medicine, a medical problem that occurs during a disease, or after a procedure or treatment. The complication may be caused by the disease, procedure, or treatment or may be unrelated to them.

cystoscope: A thin, tube-like instrument used to look inside the bladder and urethra. A cystoscope has a light and a lens for viewing and may have a tool to remove tissue.

dihydrotestosterone: A hormone made from testosterone in the prostate, testes, and certain other tissues. It is needed to develop and maintain male sex characteristics, such as facial hair, deep voice, and muscle growth. High amounts of dihydrotestosterone may increase the growth of prostate cancer and make it harder to treat. Also called androstanolone and DHT.

discharge: In medicine, a fluid that comes out of the body. Discharge can be normal or a sign of disease.

DRE (digital rectal examination): An examination in which a doctor inserts a lubricated, gloved finger into the rectum to feel for abnormalities.

duct: In medicine, a tube or vessel of the body through which fluids pass.

dutasteride: A drug used to treat symptoms of an enlarged prostate gland. It is being studied in the treatment of male hair loss and prostate cancer. Dutasteride blocks enzymes the body needs to make male sex hormones. It is a type of 5-alpha reductase inhibitor. Also called Avodart and GG745.

ejaculation: The release of semen through the penis during orgasm.

enzyme: A protein that speeds up chemical reactions in the body.

erection: When the penis temporarily gets longer, thicker, and harder. This happens because the nervous system increases the blood flow to the veins and spongy tissues of the penis.

false-positive test result: A test result that indicates that a person has a specific disease or condition when the person actually does not have the disease or condition.

family history: A record of the relationships among family members along with their medical histories. This includes current and past illnesses. A family history may show a pattern of certain diseases in a family. Also called family medical history.

(FDA) Food and Drug Administration: An agency in the U.S. federal government whose mission is to protect public health by making sure that food, cosmetics, and nutritional supplements are safe to use and truthfully labeled. The Food and Drug Administration also makes sure that drugs, medical devices, and equipment are safe and effective, and that blood for transfusions and transplant tissue are safe.

free PSA: A test that reports the percentage of free PSA (relative to total PSA) in a man's blood. Free PSA is a form of PSA that is not attached to another protein. Levels of both free and attached PSA tend to be higher in men with BPH, whereas levels of attached but not free PSA are increased in men with prostate cancer. Measuring free PSA in a man with a higher PSA level helps to tell what kind of prostate problem he has.

general anesthesia: A temporary loss of feeling and a complete loss of awareness that feels like a very deep sleep. It is caused by special drugs or other substances called anesthetics. General anesthesia keeps patients from feeling pain during surgery or other procedures.

genital: The area around male and female sex organs.

Gleason score: A system of grading prostate cancer cells based on how they look under a microscope. Gleason scores range from 2 to 10 and indicate how likely it is that a tumor will spread. A low Gleason score means the cancer cells are similar to normal prostate cells and are less likely to spread; a high Gleason score means the cancer cells are very different from normal and are more likely to spread.

groin: The area where the thigh meets the abdomen.

hyperplasia: An abnormal increase in the number of cells in an organ or tissue.

impotence: In medicine, refers to the inability to have an erection of the penis adequate for sexual intercourse. Also called erectile dysfunction.

incontinence: Inability to control the flow of urine from the bladder (urinary incontinence) or the escape of stool from the rectum (fecal incontinence).

infection: Invasion and multiplication of germs in the body. Infections can occur in any part of the body and can spread throughout the body. The germs may be bacteria, viruses, yeast, or fungi. They can cause a fever and other problems, depending on where the infection occurs. When the body's natural defense system is strong, it can often fight the germs and prevent infection. Some cancer treatments can weaken the natural defense system.

infertility: The inability to produce children.

inflammation: Redness, swelling, pain, and/or a feeling of heat in an area of the body. This is a protective reaction to injury, disease, or irritation of the tissues.

kidney: One of a pair of organs in the abdomen. Kidneys remove waste from the blood (as urine), produce erythropoietin (a substance that stimulates red blood cell production), and play a role in blood pressure regulation.

laser: A device that concentrates light into an intense, narrow beam used to cut or destroy tissue. It is used in microsurgery, photodynamic therapy, and for a variety of diagnostic purposes.

lubricant: An oily or slippery substance.

lubricated: See lubricant.

lymph node: A rounded mass of lymphatic tissue that is surrounded by a capsule of connective tissue. Lymph nodes filter lymph (lymphatic fluid), and they store lymphocytes (white blood cells). They are located along lymphatic vessels. Also called lymph gland.

medical oncologist: A doctor who specializes in diagnosing and treating cancer using chemotherapy, hormonal therapy, biological therapy, and targeted therapy. A medical oncologist often is the main health care provider for someone who has cancer. A medical oncologist also gives supportive care and may coordinate treatment given by other specialists.

metastasize: To spread from one part of the body to another. When cancer cells metastasize and form secondary tumors, the cells in the new tumor are like those in the original (primary) tumor.

nanogram: A measure of weight. One nanogram weighs a billion times less than one gram, and almost a trillion times less than a pound.

obstruction: Blockage of a passageway.

orgasm: The final part of the sex act, which involves contraction of sexual organs and a sudden release of endorphins, leading to a feeling of pleasure. In males, orgasm usually occurs with release of semen.

over-the-counter: A medicine that can be bought without a prescription (doctor's order). Examples include analgesics (pain relievers) such as aspirin and acetaminophen. Also called nonprescription and OTC.

pathologist: A doctor who identifies diseases by studying cells and tissues under a microscope.

pathology report: The description of cells and tissues made by a pathologist based on microscopic evidence, and sometimes used to make a diagnosis of a disease.

pelvis: The lower part of the belly, between the hip bones.

penis: An external male reproductive organ. It contains a tube called the urethra, which carries semen and urine to the outside of the body.

personal medical history: A collection of information about a person's health. It may include information about allergies, illnesses and surgeries, and dates and results of physical exams, tests, screenings, and immunizations. It may also include information about medicines taken and about diet and exercise. Also called personal health record and personal history.

positive test result: A test result that reveals the presence of a specific disease or condition for which the test is being done.

precancerous: Describes a condition that may (or is likely to) become cancer. Also called premalignant.

prescription: A doctor's order for medicine or another intervention.

prostate: A gland in the male reproductive system. The prostate surrounds the part of the urethra (the tube that empties the bladder) just below the bladder, and produces a fluid that forms part of the semen.

prostate cancer: Cancer that forms in tissues of the prostate (a gland in the male reproductive system found below the bladder and in front of the rectum). Prostate cancer usually occurs in older men.

prostatitis: Inflammation of the prostate gland.

protein: A molecule made up of amino acids that are needed for the body to function properly. Proteins are the basis of body structures such as skin and hair and of substances such as enzymes, cytokines, and antibodies.

PSA (prostate-specific antigen): A substance produced by the prostate that may be found in an increased amount in the blood of men who have prostate cancer, benign prostatic hyperplasia, or infection or inflammation of the prostate.

PSA test: A blood test to measure PSA, a substance produced by prostate gland cells. This level rises when there is a problem with the prostate gland. But the PSA test cannot tell whether the problem is cancer or another condition.

radiation oncologist: A doctor who specializes in using radiation to treat cancer.

rectal: By or having to do with the rectum.

rectum: The last several inches of the large intestine, ending at the anus.

reproductive system: The organs involved in producing offspring. In women, this system includes the ovaries, the fallopian tubes, the uterus (womb), the cervix, and the vagina (birth canal). In men, it includes the prostate, the testes, and the penis.

risk factor: Something that may increase the chance of developing a disease. Some examples of risk factors for cancer include age, a family history of certain cancers, use of tobacco products, certain eating habits, obesity, lack of exercise, exposure to radiation or other cancer-causing agents, and certain genetic changes.

recurrence: Cancer that has recurred (come back), usually after a period of time during which the cancer could not be detected. The cancer may come back to the same place as the original (primary) tumor or to another place in the body. Also called recurrent cancer.

screening: Checking for disease when there are no symptoms. Since screening may find diseases at an early stage, there may be a better chance of curing the disease. Examples of cancer screening tests are the mammogram (breast), colonoscopy (colon), Pap smear (cervix), and PSA blood level and digital rectal exam (prostate). Screening can also include checking for a person's risk of developing an inherited disease by doing a genetic test.

scrotum: In men, the external sac that contains the testicles.

semen: The fluid that is released through the penis during orgasm. Semen is made up of sperm from the testicles and fluid from the prostate and other sex glands.

side effect: A problem that occurs when treatment affects healthy tissues or organs. Some common side effects of cancer treatment are fatigue, pain, nausea, vomiting, decreased blood cell counts, hair loss, and mouth sores.

skin cancer: Cancer that forms in tissues of the skin. There are several types of skin cancer. Skin cancer that forms in melanocytes (skin cells that make pigment) is called melanoma. Skin cancer that forms in basal cells (small, round cells in the base of the outer layer of skin) is called basal cell carcinoma. Skin cancer that forms in squamous cells (flat cells that form the surface of the skin) is called squamous cell carcinoma. Skin cancer that forms in neuroendocrine cells (cells that release hormones in response to signals from the nervous system) is called neuroendocrine carcinoma of the skin. Most skin cancers form in older people on parts of the body exposed to the sun or in people who have weakened immune systems.

sperm: The male reproductive cell, formed in the testicle. A sperm joins with an egg to form an embryo.

spinal block: A type of anesthesia that numbs the lower half of the body.

stage: The extent of a cancer in the body. Staging is usually based on the size of the tumor, whether lymph nodes contain cancer, and whether the cancer has spread from the original site to other parts of the body.

surgery: A procedure to remove or repair a part of the body or to find out whether disease is present. An operation.

symptom: An indication that a person has a condition or disease. Some examples of symptoms are headache, fever, fatigue, nausea, vomiting, and pain.

testicle: One of two egg-shaped glands inside the scrotum that produce sperm and male hormones. Also called testis.

testosterone: A hormone made mainly in the testes (part of the male reproductive system). It is needed to develop and maintain male sex characteristics, such as facial hair, deep voice, and muscle growth. Testosterone may also be made in the laboratory and is used to treat certain medical conditions.

tissue: A group or layer of cells that work together to perform a specific function.

tumor: An abnormal mass of tissue that results when cells divide more than they should or do not die when they should. Tumors may be benign (not cancer) or malignant (cancer). Also called neoplasm.

urethra: The tube through which urine leaves the body. It empties urine from the bladder.

urinary: Having to do with urine or the organs of the body that produce and get rid of urine.

urinary tract: The organs of the body that produce and discharge urine. These include the kidneys, ureters, bladder, and urethra.

urine: Fluid containing water and waste products. Urine is made by the kidneys, stored in the bladder, and leaves the body through the urethra.

urologic oncologist: A doctor who specializes in treating cancers of the urinary system and the male reproductive system.

urologist: A doctor who specializes in diseases of the urinary organs in females and the urinary and sex organs in males.

watchful waiting: Closely monitoring a patient's condition but withholding treatment until symptoms appear or change. Also called active surveillance, expectant management, and observation.

For more information,
or to order free copies
of this booklet:

Call 1-800-4-CANCER

(1-800-422-6237)

or visit www.cancer.gov

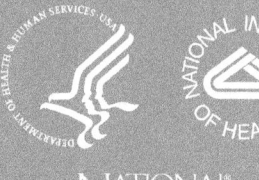

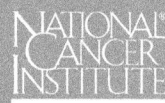

NIH Publication No. 11-4303
Reprinted August 2011